I0768018

THE ART OF
CLONING PERFUME

HOW TO RECREATE FAMOUS PERFUMES WITH ESSENTIAL OILS

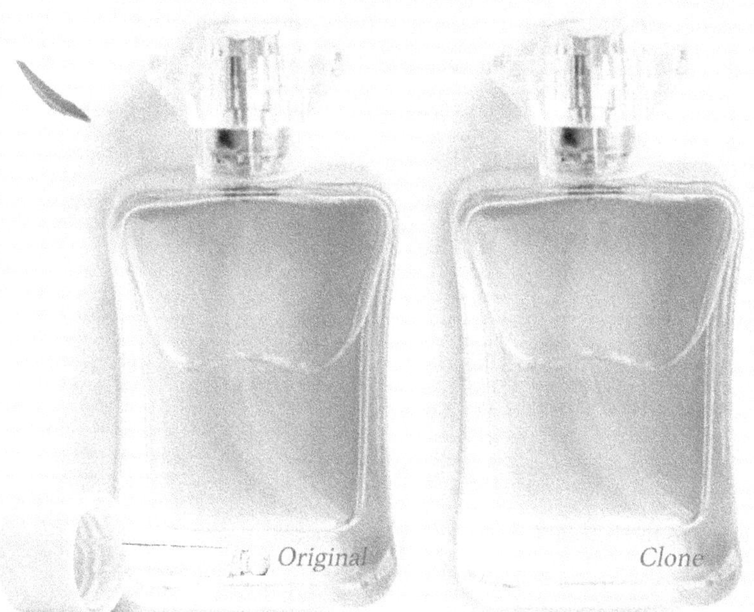

REBECCA PARK TOTILO

The Art of Cloning Perfume
How to Recreate Famous Perfumes with Essential Oils

The Natural Perfume Series — Book Three

Copyright © 2026. Rebecca Park Totilo

All rights reserved. No part of this book may be reproduced or transmitted in any form or by any means—electronic, mechanical, photocopy, recording, or otherwise—without the written permission of the copyright holder, except as provided by USA copyright law.

Educational Scope and Limitations
This book is intended as an educational guide to analytical perfume cloning. It does not reproduce proprietary formulas or support commercial replication. Its purpose is to demonstrate how structural analysis, evaluation, and refinement function within a disciplined cloning framework, and to provide a study model that can be applied to other fragrances.

All fragrance names mentioned in this book are the property of their respective trademark holders and are referenced solely for educational and comparative purposes.

Printed in the United States of America.
Published by Rebecca at the Well Foundation.
Paperback ISBN: 979-8-9937841-3-7
Electronic ISBN: 979-8-9937841-4-4

Contents

Chapter 1: Perfume Cloning: Structure and Method 1

❖ From Duplication to Interpretation 1
❖ Cloning as a Method of Study 2
❖ The Art of Deconstruction 3
❖ The Challenge and the Discipline of Cloning 3
❖ Essential Oils as Analytical Tools 4
❖ Why Clone at All? 4
❖ A Framework for the Chapters Ahead 5
❖ How to Use This Book 5

Chapter 2: Researching Commercial Perfumes for Cloning 7

❖ Steps to Identify Accords in Popular Perfumes 8
❖ Relevant Information 9

Chapter 3: Fragrance Families and Perfume Structure 11

❖ The Four Primary Fragrance Families (Cloning Perspective) 11
❖ Other Fragrance Families as Cloning Shortcuts 13
❖ Common Fragrance Families and Their Characteristics 14
❖ Why Fragrance Families Matter in Perfume Cloning 15

Chapter 4: imits, Ethics, and Interpretation in Fragrance Cloning 17

❖ Understanding the Limits of Replication 18
❖ Mainstream Versus Niche Structures 18
❖ From Reconstruction to Interpretation 19

❖ Practical Reference Material 19
❖ Ethical Considerations 20
❖ Legality vs. Integrity 20
❖ Transparency with Clients 20

Chapter 5: Scent Profiling for Fragrance Analysis **22**
❖ Breaking Down a Fragrance for Analysis 22
❖ Analytical Techniques for Scent Profiling 23
❖ How to Identify Top, Heart, and Base Notes in a Perfume 25
❖ Observed Structural Emphasis 27
❖ From Profiling to Material Selection 31

Chapter 6: Choosing the Right Essential Oils for Cloning **33**
❖ Reconstructing the Scent with Essential Oils 34
❖ Balancing and Refining the Clone Over Time 35
❖ Selecting Essential Oils to Match Popular Scent Profiles 35
❖ Substituting Natural Ingredients for Synthetics 37
❖ Decoding the Original Scent Profile 39
❖ Understanding Variations in Essential Oil Quality 42
❖ Practical Guidance for Cloning with Natural Materials 43
❖ Complete Clone Walkthrough 44
❖ Initial Smell Evaluation 45
❖ Pyramid Interpretation 45
❖ Structural Analysis 47
❖ Material Selection 47
❖ First Blend 49
❖ Evaluation 51
❖ Adjustment 51
❖ Purpose of the Walkthrough 52

Chapter 7: Natural Material Approximation **53**
❖ The Role of Approximation in Natural Cloning 53
❖ Example: Natural Approximation of an Oriental-Spicy Structure 54
❖ Addressing the Absence of Synthetic Effects 55
❖ Evaluating Natural Approximations 55

Chapter 8: Blending Techniques for Fragrance Cloning................................57

❖ Blending by Note...57

❖ Blending by Accord: Structural Frameworks in Fragrance Cloning ... 60

❖ Blending by Aromatic Group 64

❖ Common Aromatic Group Frameworks.......................67

❖ Blending for Longevity and Sillage 68

Chapter 9: From Analysis to Reconstruction...70

❖ Instructions for Making a Clone Perfume.....................70

❖ Making Your Own Signature Scent from a Clone 73

❖ Experimenting with New Notes and Accords.................74

❖ Development Process for the Clone...............................75

❖ Natural Chanel No. 5–Inspired Fragrance Clone...........78

Chapter 10: Testing and Perfecting Your Perfume Clone...............................81

❖ Evaluating Scent Development Over Time 81

❖ Adjusting Proportions and Ratios 82

Chapter 11: Common Issues and How to Fix Them 85

❖ Keep Blending Notes..90

Appendix A: Natural Substitutes for Synthetic Notes 91

❖ Fruity Notes 91

❖ Gourmand Notes...92

❖ Floral & Green Notes...93

❖ Wood, Resin & Earth Notes 94

❖ Fresh, Airy & Marine Notes 95

❖ Spice, Balsam & Exotic Notes 96

❖ Floral Family 96

❖ Citrus Family 97

❖ Woody Family...98

❖ Gourmand Family 98

❖ Fresh/Oceanic Family 99

❖ Oriental/Resinous Family 99

Appendix B: Famous Perfume Accords...100

Appendix C: All-Natural Perfume Clone Recipes..103

❖ Chanel No. 5–Inspired (Classic Aldehydic Floral)..................................104
❖ Dior Sauvage-Inspired (Fresh Spicy Woody)..105
❖ Black Orchid-Inspired (Oriental Floral Gourmand)............................106
❖ Light Blue-Inspired (Citrus Fruity Woody)...107
❖ Aventus-Inspired (Fruity Chypre)..108
❖ Black Opium-Inspired (Gourmand Oriental).......................................109
❖ La Vie Est Belle-Inspired (Fruity Floral Gourmand).........................110

CHAPTER 1
Perfume Cloning:
Structure and Method

Perfume unfolds over time. It announces itself, settles into a character, and leaves an impression that lingers long after the first moment. This progression is deliberate, shaped by material choice, proportion, and timing rather than chance.

In this book, perfume cloning is used to learn how that progression is built. You will study how established fragrances are organized, observe how they change across wear, and reconstruct their structure using natural materials. The goal is not imitation, but understanding—developing the ability to recognize balance, transition, and emphasis, and use those principles with confidence in your own work.

From Duplication to Interpretation

Throughout history, perfumers have attempted to recreate costly fragrances—sometimes out of admiration, sometimes to meet popular demand. What has changed is not the act itself, but the method and intention behind it.

In commercial perfumery, duplication typically relies on molecular analysis and synthetic reconstruction. Fragrances are reverse-engineered by isolating aroma chemicals and reassembling them into formulas designed for consistency, projection, and scalability. These duplicates are often produced at scale and marketed as alternatives to the original.

Natural perfume cloning operates under a fundamentally different approach. Rather than pursuing molecular equivalence, the natural perfumer works with essential oils, absolutes, resins, and other botanical materials to **interpret** a fragrance's structure and behavior. The objective is not exact replication, but functional resemblance—capturing the balance, progression, and emotional signature of a scent using materials derived from nature.

Cloning as a Method of Study

In this book, cloning is treated as a method of study. By deconstructing existing fragrances, the natural perfumer learns how a scent is organized, how its identity is established, and how it evolves on the skin. Cloning exposes the internal structure of perfume—what leads, what supports, and what anchors a composition over time.

Rather than teaching how to build a fragrance from a blank slate, this approach teaches how to study an existing one—observing its progression, identifying its defining elements, and reconstructing its structure using natural materials. The emphasis is not on note lists or marketing descriptions, but on structure, balance, and behavior.

The Art of Deconstruction

At its core, perfume cloning is an act of deconstruction. It involves breaking a fragrance into its functional layers—its opening impression, its defining heart, and its lasting base—while paying close attention to accords, transitions, and proportional relationships.

This process requires more than identifying notes printed on a label. It demands an attentive nose, an understanding of fragrance structure, and the ability to perceive subtle shifts as a scent evolves. Through deconstruction, perfume moves from the abstract to the intelligible, revealing an underlying framework that can be studied and translated.

The Challenge and the Discipline of Cloning

Fragrance cloning with natural materials is both rewarding and complex. Commercial perfumes often rely on proprietary formulas and synthetic materials that cannot be duplicated using natural ingredients alone. Individual perception and skin chemistry further influence how a fragrance performs. For these reasons, successful cloning is not about precision copying, but about disciplined interpretation.

The challenge lies in capturing a fragrance's essence—its weight and direction—while working within the expressive limits of natural materials. This requires restraint, structural awareness, and a willingness to prioritize coherence over literal accuracy.

Essential Oils as Analytical Tools

Essential oils form the foundation of natural perfume cloning. Unlike synthetic aroma chemicals designed for uniformity and control, essential oils are complex botanical extracts shaped by soil, climate, and time. Each oil contains multiple aromatic facets that emerge and recede as a fragrance develops.

While not every synthetic effect has a direct natural equivalent, skilled blending allows the natural perfumer to suggest familiar qualities—brightness, warmth, softness, depth—through carefully constructed accords. Working with essential oils encourages a responsive, evaluative approach to perfume creation, prioritizing balance and evolution over static effects.

In this context, essential oils are not merely ingredients; they are analytical tools. They demonstrate how structure behaves in the presence of material complexity.

Why Clone at All?

Fragrance cloning develops analytical skill. By studying how established perfumes are constructed, the perfumer learns to recognize structure, proportion, and material function beyond surface impressions.

Because many contemporary fragrances rely on synthetic effects without direct natural equivalents, cloning with essential oils requires interpretation rather than replication. This process strengthens sensory awareness and refines structural judgment, allowing perfume to be understood as a system that can be observed, analyzed, and re-created with intention.

A Framework for the Chapters Ahead

This book presents a clear, methodical approach to perfume cloning as an analytical practice. You will progress from research and structural analysis into material selection, reconstruction, and refinement, with an emphasis on understanding rather than memorization.

By studying how fragrances are built, how they behave over time, and how their structure can be translated using natural materials, you develop the ability to work like a perfumer—observing, evaluating, adjusting, and creating with intention.

How to Use This Book

This book is designed to be read progressively, though not strictly linearly. Perfume cloning is a cumulative skill, and many sections are meant to be revisited as your experience deepens. Early chapters establish the analytical frameworks and vocabulary that are applied repeatedly throughout later work.

Throughout this text, certain terms are used to describe structural or functional effects rather than specific ingredients. For example, *aldehydic* refers to a perceived effect—sparkle, lift, diffusion, and clean brightness—rather than the presence of synthetic aldehyde molecules. When working with natural materials, these effects are approached through structure and material behavior rather than chemical replication.

This is not a recipe collection or a guide to exact duplication. Instead, it presents a structured method for studying existing perfumes and translating their behavior using natural materials. As you move through the exercises and examples, expect to shift between chapters; skill develops through observation, comparison, and refinement over time.

With this analytical framework in place, the next step is research—learning how to gather and interpret publicly available information about commercial perfumes to support accurate structural analysis.

Chapter 2
Researching Commercial Perfumes for Cloning

Cloning a perfume with essential oils begins with research into the original fragrance. Before any smelling, blending, or reconstruction takes place, the natural perfumer gathers publicly available information describing how the fragrance is structured and perceived. Public fragrance databases such as Fragrantica and Basenotes are used as reference tools to support structural analysis, not as authoritative sources for formulas or exact ingredient compositions.

This chapter explains how to locate a fragrance, review its published note pyramid, identify its fragrance family and dominant accords, examine performance data such as longevity and sillage, and extract relevant insights from user reviews and perfumer information. The goal of this chapter is documentation—collecting structured reference data that will later support accurate analysis and reconstruction.

Steps to Identify Accords in Popular Perfumes

1. **Search for the Fragrance.**

   Open your web browser and go to Fragrantica or Basenotes. Use the site's search function to enter the name of the fragrance you wish to analyze.

2. **Review the Fragrance Pyramid.**

   Look for the fragrance pyramid, which breaks down a perfume's top, heart (middle), and base notes. This can often be found on the perfume's official website or on the aforementioned fragrance databases.

3. **Analyze the Listed Notes.**

   Identify the listed notes and categorize them into top, middle, and base notes. This will help you understand the fragrance's structure.

4. **Identify Common Accords.**

   Based on the notes, you can identify common accords. For example, if the perfume lists bergamot, lemon, and orange in the top notes, this typically indicates a citrus accord. If it lists jasmine, rose, and ylang ylang in the middle notes, it likely has a floral accord.

5. **Read Reviews and User Feedback.**

   Read user reviews and expert descriptions to identify recurring patterns. Pay attention to how the fragrance is commonly characterized (for example, woody, floral, oriental, or aquatic), as these terms often point to dominant accords. Note comments on longevity and sillage to understand performance, and review discussion sections to observe shared perceptions and interpretive trends.

6. **Note the Perfumer.**

The page will also list the perfumer who created the fragrance, which can provide additional context about stylistic influences. Take notes on the details that are most relevant to your clone project, as this information will guide your structural analysis and reconstruction.

7. **Consult Perfume Community Forums.**

Consult perfume community discussions on platforms such as Fragrantica or Basenotes to review longer-form analyses, comparisons, and differing interpretations. These conversations often reveal nuanced observations about structure, balance, and evolution that are not captured in standard note listings or summaries.

Relevant Information

Perfume Pyramid: A visual or textual representation showing the hierarchy of the top, middle, and base notes

Perfumer: The name of the person who created the fragrance; knowing the perfumer can help you understand the style and common ingredients they use

Fragrance Family: The category or family the fragrance belongs to (e.g., floral, oriental, woody, fresh); this helps you understand the overall character of the scent

Accords: Dominant characteristics of the fragrance (e.g., spicy, powdery, sweet)

Longevity and Sillage: Longevity is how long the fragrance lasts on the skin; sillage is the trail left by the fragrance, or how far the scent diffuses around the wearer

User Commentary on Performance and Perception: Read what other users have to say about the fragrance; this can provide insights into how the fragrance performs and is perceived by others

Release Year: The year the fragrance was launched; this can provide context regarding its style and trends at the time

CHAPTER 3
Fragrance Families and Perfume Structure

In perfume cloning, fragrance families are used as analytical reference points rather than stylistic categories. Identifying a fragrance's dominant family helps clarify its overall direction, weight, and emphasis before individual materials are considered. Because essential oils can shift roles depending on proportion and context, family classification in cloning functions as a diagnostic tool rather than a fixed label.

The Four Primary Fragrance Families (Cloning Perspective)

In perfume cloning, the four primary fragrance families—floral, amber (oriental), woody, and fresh—are used to identify which family dominates a fragrance, not to describe scent styles. Determining which family anchors a fragrance helps predict weight, diffusion, and where synthetic effects are likely contributing to performance characteristics.

Floral-dominant structures typically define the heart of a fragrance and carry its recognizability. Florals often require structural support to prevent collapse or distortion during drydown.

Common floral materials used for structural reconstruction: rose, jasmine, neroli, ylang ylang, lavender, roman chamomile, geranium.

Amber (Oriental) structures contribute warmth, density, and persistence. These structures frequently rely on synthetic fixatives in commercial perfumes, making them critical areas for natural substitution and accord-building.

Common amber materials used for structural reconstruction: vanilla absolute, benzoin, frankincense, myrrh, patchouli, labdanum, peru balsam.

Woody structures function as anchors and transitional frameworks. In cloning, woods are often responsible for longevity and cohesion, but can easily overpower if not proportioned carefully.

Common woody materials used for structure: sandalwood or amyris, cedarwood (atlas or virginia), vetiver, patchouli, guaiacwood.

Fresh structures dominate openings and diffusion, but are the least stable when translated with essential oils. These structures often require reinforcement to maintain lift without rapid fading.

Common fresh materials used for opening effects: citrus oils (bergamot, lemon, grapefruit, lime, sweet orange, petitgrain), green notes (galbanum, violet leaf, basil), and select materials that suggest aquatic or fruity effects.

In cloning work, these families should be treated as analytical reference points. They help identify where emphasis exists in the original composition, where natural materials will need reinforcement, and where interpretive construction is required to preserve recognizability over time.

Other Fragrance Families as Cloning Shortcuts

Beyond primary family identification, secondary and hybrid families function as **refinement tools** during fragrance deconstruction. Once the dominant structure is recognized, these families help clarify nuance—such as sweetness, dryness, density, or diffusion—that may not be obvious from top-line analysis alone.

In cloning, hybrid family identification (e.g., floral-amber, woody-fresh, gourmand-oriental) helps narrow functional requirements rather than specific ingredients. This allows the natural perfumer to anticipate where synthetic effects are shaping performance and where natural accords will be needed to support or extend those effects.

Because commercial fragrances often shift family emphasis as they develop, family roles should be assessed dynamically rather than fixed at first impression. A material may function as a driver at one stage and a modifier or bridge at another. For this reason, secondary families are best used to confirm structural decisions and guide supportive construction as the cloning process develops.

Fragrances are commonly categorized into families based on their dominant aromatic theme. Identifying the family of a perfume during analysis can provide insight into its underlying structure and the types of materials likely contributing to its character.

The table below summarizes common fragrance families, their general traits, and the natural materials frequently associated with each category. These categories are included as reference context and should be interpreted structurally rather than stylistically when cloning.

Common Fragrance Families and Their Characteristics

The following families include both primary and secondary categories and are provided as structural reference rather than hierarchical classification.

Family	Characteristics	Essential Oils Commonly Used
Citrus	bright, fresh, energetic	lemon, bergamot, grapefruit, petitgrain
Floral	soft, romantic, feminine	rose, jasmine, ylang ylang, neroli
Amber (Oriental)	warm, spicy, exotic	vanilla, patchouli, myrrh, clove

Family	Characteristics	Essential Oils Commonly Used
Woody	dry, smooth, grounding	sandalwood, cedarwood, vetiver
Aromatic	herbal, clean, invigorating	lavender, sage, rosemary, basil
Chypre	mossy, earthy, complex	bergamot, oakmoss, patchouli, labdanum
Fougère	barbershop, classic masculine	lavender, geranium, tonka bean, oakmoss
Gourmand	edible, sweet, cozy	vanilla, benzoin, cocoa absolute
Leather	smoky, animalic, bold	birch tar, styrax, cistus labdanum

Understanding these categories helps you deconstruct the perfume's style and reconstruct it more fully. For instance, if you're cloning a fougère fragrance, you know you'll likely need lavender, oakmoss, and a coumarin-rich note like tonka or sweet hay.

Why Fragrance Families Matter in Perfume Cloning

Identifying a fragrance's dominant family helps clarify its underlying structure, weight, and direction before individual materials are considered. This allows the natural perfumer to focus on how a scent is organized and supported over time, rather than relying on note lists or marketing descriptions.

Because many commercial perfumes blend multiple families or shift family emphasis as they develop, classification is most useful for recognizing structural dominance and synthetic influence. In cloning, this information guides material selection, proportion, and the construction of supporting accords needed to translate the original fragrance using natural materials.

Used correctly, fragrance families act as a structural guide—helping the natural perfumer interpret complexity, anticipate challenges, and reconstruct a fragrance with clarity and intention rather than guesswork.

CHAPTER 4
Limits, Ethics, and Interpretation in Fragrance Cloning

Fragrance cloning is a structured analytical practice with clear boundaries. While earlier chapters focused on reconstruction—identifying accords, balance, and performance—this chapter clarifies the limits of cloning and how it should be used responsibly within professional perfumery study. This chapter defines the scope and proper use of the cloning process.

By deconstructing an existing perfume and reconstructing its form, the natural perfumer gains insight into proportion, balance, material behavior, and overall structure. Successful cloning reproduces how a fragrance opens, develops, and dries down over time.

Understanding the Limits of Replication

Not all perfumes can be cloned with equal precision. Commercial fragrances often rely on proprietary aroma chemicals, captive molecules, or specialized extraction methods that are unavailable outside industrial settings, and regulatory restrictions or material availability may further limit direct substitution. When working primarily with natural materials, these constraints become more pronounced.

In these cases, cloning focuses on approximation. The natural perfumer must determine which aspects of the perfume are essential to its identity and which can be interpreted. Cloning focuses on recreating a fragrance's recognizable character and development using natural materials.

Mainstream Versus Niche Structures

Mainstream perfumes are often built around familiar, repeatable frameworks designed for consistency, diffusion, and broad appeal. These structures are typically easier to analyze and reconstruct because they rely on standardized proportions and widely used accords. Niche and artisan perfumes, by contrast, may emphasize texture, rawness, or unconventional balance, and may be built around a single dominant material, a nontraditional accord, or a deliberately uneven evolution.

When analyzing niche or artisan fragrances, cloning shifts from duplication to interpretation. The natural perfumer must identify what defines the perfume's presence, such as its weight, contrast, or overall structural character. Attempting to force such perfumes into conventional cloning templates can obscure their intent. In these cases, cloning becomes a study in restraint, clarifying what should be preserved rather than replicated.

From Reconstruction to Interpretation

Once a perfume's structure has been analyzed and approximated, the natural perfumer has a functional reference point. It is important to distinguish between reconstruction and interpretation: reconstruction seeks alignment with the original fragrance, while interpretation applies insights gained through cloning to explore related ideas.

This book focuses on reconstruction. Any movement beyond that—toward personalization, variation, or bespoke creation—constitutes a separate discipline with distinct evaluation criteria. Understanding where cloning ends maintains clarity of purpose and preserves the technical integrity of the process.

Practical Reference Material

Detailed clone formulas, ingredient substitutions, and inspired variations are included only as reference material and are not part of the main cloning method presented in this book. Where useful, such materials are included in the appendix as optional reference examples. These references are provided for study and should not be understood as part of the primary analytical method presented in the text.

Ethical Considerations

Approached responsibly, perfume cloning is an educational practice. Recreating fragrances for personal study or technical exploration is generally accepted when done with respect for original creators and without claims of brand association. This book emphasizes ethical interpretation rather than imitation, encouraging readers to learn from existing perfumes while developing informed and original work.

Legality vs. Integrity

In most countries, perfumes are not protected under copyright law. This means it is technically legal to replicate a scent, but legality and ethics are not the same.

Consider the following points:

- Are you selling a product that could be confused with the original?
- Are you giving appropriate attribution (for example, "inspired by," not "the same as")?
- Are you respecting the artistry of the original work?

Transparency with Clients

If you are creating bespoke fragrances for others, be clear about whether a blend is a clone or inspired by a known perfume. Clients may request a scent similar to a well-known perfume, but it is your responsibility to explain how your version differs and to set appropriate expectations.

Having established the boundaries, limitations, and ethical context of fragrance cloning, the focus now shifts from conceptual understanding to applied sensory analysis. Cloning cannot proceed through research or structural theory alone; it requires direct engagement with the perfume itself.

The next chapter introduces scent profiling as a practical discipline, training the nose to observe dominance, transitions, and balance over time. This analytical step forms the foundation for accurate reconstruction using natural materials.

CHAPTER 5

Scent Profiling for Fragrance Analysis

———

This chapter moves from structural theory into applied analysis, focusing on how finished perfumes are evaluated through sensory observation and timed wear. Building on concepts of structure, balance, and performance established earlier, the goal is to develop practical skills for identifying dominance, transitions, and weaknesses within an existing composition. Rather than redefining fragrance components, the focus is on recognizing structural behavior in real time as a foundation for accurate reconstruction using natural materials.

Breaking Down a Fragrance for Analysis

To begin cloning a perfume, you must first deconstruct it. This doesn't require a gas chromatograph; it requires time, patience, and a well-trained nose. Spray a sample of the perfume onto a blotter or strip and begin by analyzing the first few moments—this is the opening/top phase. What do you detect first? Is it citrusy, green, fruity? Record your impressions immediately, as top notes fade quickly.

After 15–20 minutes, revisit the strip. Now you are in the heart of the fragrance—the middle note territory. Floral, herbal, or spicy elements may become more apparent. Common indicators at this stage may include jasmine, rose, lavender, or cardamom.

.Finally, after an hour or more, assess the base notes. The foundation of any perfume is found here: woods, resins, musks, or balsamic tones that linger. These can include vetiver, patchouli, benzoin, myrrh, or labdanum. By carefully separating your analysis into these three phases, you can begin to sketch a vertical profile of the perfume you are analyzing for reconstruction.

At this stage, observations should be documented for later use during reconstruction rather than translated directly into a formula. Organize what you observe by phase—opening, heart, and base—and note relative dominance (primary, supporting, trace), transitions, and any gaps or collapses over time. The more dominant a feature is in the original perfume, the more structural emphasis it will require in your clone, but exact proportions should be determined only after repeated wear tests and comparative evaluation.

Analytical Techniques for Scent Profiling

Profiling a perfume combines structured analysis with trained sensory observation. Use the following techniques to improve your analysis skills:

1. The Smell + Describe Method

- Smell the perfume and write down every impression—even if it is abstract.
- Example: fresh cut grass, powdery, lemon candy, or warm spice.
- Then note which natural materials may correspond to these impressions, without committing to specific selections.

2. Fragrance Strip Comparisons

- Use individual essential oil blotters to compare and isolate a match.
- Line them up next to your target perfume and smell them side by side.
- Consider whether the material corresponds to any element perceived in the original perfume.

3. Triangle Charting

- Sketch a triangle and label each layer (top, heart, base).
- As you analyze, place the perceived scent elements into each layer.
- This creates a visual representation of the perfume's structure.

4. Digital and Community Tools

- Use reference databases such as Fragrantica, Basenotes, or Parfumo.
- Look up the perfume you are analyzing for cloning:

- Listed notes (official and user-voted)
- Fragrance family
- Performance and longevity reports

Caution: These sites often include synthetic ingredients, so the task is to translate the note list into natural counterparts. For example:

- "White musk" might become ambrette seed CO_2.
- "Marine accord" may be approximated using seaweed absolute or cypress.

How to Identify Top, Heart, and Base Notes in a Perfume

The first step in cloning a perfume is recognizing its structure as it unfolds through the opening, development, and drydown.

Step-by-Step Sensory Breakdown

1. **Apply the perfume to a strip.**

   Use a fragrance blotter. Allow the perfume to develop without interference.

2. **Observe the first 0–10 minutes (top notes).**

   These notes are sharp, fresh, and light—often citrus, herbs, or bright spices. Write down your impressions immediately.

3. **Wait 10–30 minutes (heart notes).**

   As the top fades, you may notice floral, fruity, or spicy notes. These notes define the fragrance's core theme.

4. **Observe the drydown after 1–3 hours (base notes).**

   Base notes include woods, resins, musks, and rich balsamics. They anchor the fragrance and linger longest.

Use this timeline to build a three-part description of the perfume. For more accurate reconstruction, repeat the analysis across several wears on both blotter and skin, and note how the perfume shifts over time, with temperature, and with application method.

Case Study Overview

To illustrate how fragrance structure can be analyzed and translated into a reconstruction strategy, the following example examines a well-known commercial perfume. The fragrance selected for this case study is Estée Lauder's *Youth-Dew*, a classic oriental-spicy composition recognized for its rich balsamic base, pronounced spice heart, and citrus opening with an aldehydic lift. Its bold, layered construction makes it particularly well-suited for instructional study because deviations in balance or structure are easy to detect during evaluation. The objective of this case study is to:

- Identify the **framework** of the original perfume
- Select materials that perform **similar functional roles**
- Evaluate **structural development**, weight, and persistence
- Address areas of **structural divergence** for correction

Observed Structural Emphasis

Instead of relying on marketing descriptions or note lists, the fragrance should first be evaluated through timed observation. In the case of *Youth-Dew*, the structure can be summarized as follows:

- **Top:** Citrus brightness reinforced by aldehydic effect and supported by warm spice
- **Heart:** Dense floral-spice core with pronounced clove and cinnamon character
- **Base:** Heavy balsamic and resinous foundation with vanilla, patchouli, moss, and incense-like depth

The fragrance places significant emphasis on the **base structure**, which dominates the drydown and accounts for much of its longevity and recognizable identity.

Analytical Weight Distribution

The following example illustrates an initial test structure for exploring alignment with an original perfume. Rather than presenting a finished formula, it highlights how emphasis may be distributed across the opening, heart, and base to reflect the observed character of the original scent. Percentages are provided to illustrate proportional balance rather than prescribe a fixed recipe.

- **Top Structure (approx. 25–30%)**
  Citrus materials supported by light aldehydic lift or other diffusive components

- **Heart Structure (approx. 45–50%)**

  Warm spices and florals form the core identity

- **Base Structure (approx. 20–25%)**

  Balsams, resins, woods, and fixative materials anchoring the composition

This breakdown shows where the fragrance puts its weight—what dominates the opening, what defines the scent, and what persists—so you have a clear structural target before you begin blending.

Applying the Analysis: Youth-Dew Inspired Reconstruction

With the structural profile established, the next step is to translate the fragrance's observed behavior into a reconstruction strategy using natural materials. The goal is not to reproduce the formula of the original perfume, but to approximate its character—the relationship between the bright opening, the dense spicy heart, and the heavy balsamic base that defines the scent. Based on the earlier analytical weight distribution, the reconstruction can begin with a structure that emphasizes a substantial heart supported by a warm, persistent base.

Example Structural Approach:

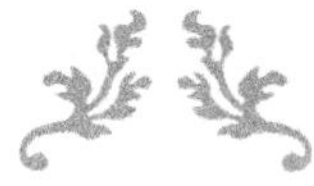

TOP STRUCTURE
(25–30%)

Citrus lift with
aldehydic-style brightness

Bergamot
Lemon or Sweet Orange
Litsea Cubeba / Lemongrass
(aldehydic effect)

HEART
STRUCTURE (45–50%)

Dense floral-spice core of
the fragrance

Clove
Cinnamon Leaf
Cardamom
Jasmine Absolute
Ylang Ylang or Rose

BASE STRUCTURE (20–25%)

Heavy
balsamic-resinous foundation

Patchouli
Labdanum
Benzoin
Frankincense or Myrrh
Vanilla Absolute
(supporting warmth)

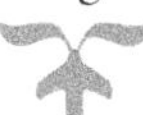

Top Structure
(approximately 25–30%)

The opening of Youth-Dew presents a citrus brightness supported by aldehydic lift. In natural reconstruction, this effect can be approximated using bergamot, sweet orange, or lemon, supported by litsea cubeba or lemongrass to create a sparkling, slightly sharp opening.

Heart Structure
(approximately 45–50%)

The defining character of the fragrance emerges in the heart, where warm spice blends with floral richness. A natural reconstruction might emphasize clove, cinnamon leaf, or cardamom, supported by florals such as jasmine absolute, ylang ylang, or rose. These materials recreate the dense, spicy-floral core that gives the fragrance its recognizable identity.

Base Structure (approximately 20–25%)

The base of *Youth-Dew* is heavy and persistent, dominated by balsams, resins, and woods. Natural reconstruction may rely on patchouli, labdanum, benzoin, frankincense, or myrrh to create a deep, resinous drydown. A small amount of vanilla absolute can reinforce the warm sweetness associated with the original composition.

This structural translation provides a practical framework for beginning a reconstruction trial. The exact proportions should be determined through iterative blending and comparative testing against the original fragrance, adjusting the balance of citrus brightness, spice density, and balsamic depth until the clone reflects the same general progression and weight.

Left Figure: Structural translation of Estée Lauder *Youth-Dew* for natural material reconstruction.

The diagram illustrates how the fragrance's observed analytical weight can be translated into a practical reconstruction strategy using essential oils and natural aromatic materials.

Material Selection Strategy

The materials in this example are chosen for the roles they play in the fragrance. Each material serves a structural purpose within the formula, such as diffusion, warmth, fixation, or depth. Where proprietary materials are unavailable, comparable alternatives are used to recreate the same effect.

Key considerations during selection include:

- Volatility and evaporation rate
- Contribution to warmth, spice, or balsamic depth
- Ability to support longevity and cohesion

Evaluation and Iteration

Once blended, the formula should be evaluated alongside the original fragrance at multiple time intervals. Key evaluation questions include:

- Does the opening deliver similar brightness and warmth?
- Does the heart maintain sufficient density and spice character?
- Does the base provide appropriate persistence and weight over time?

Any deviations are addressed by adjusting the structure rather than chasing individual notes. For example, a weak drydown indicates insufficient base weight, while an overly sharp opening suggests excessive volatility or imbalance in diffusive materials.

Plan to revise the blend multiple times, evaluating each version independently to assess structural development.

From Profiling to Material Selection

Once a fragrance has been profiled through structured observation, its reconstruction depends on the choice of materials.

Analysis reveals what the perfume does; material selection determines how closely that behavior can be translated using natural aromatics.

CHAPTER 6
Choosing the Right Essential Oils for Cloning

Fragrance cloning begins by breaking a perfume into its structural components—notes, accords, and proportional balance—and rebuilding that structure using comparable aromatic materials. Success depends on careful observation, familiarity with fragrance architecture, and the ability to recognize how individual materials contribute to the perfume's overall character.

When working with essential oils, cloning becomes a careful balancing process that integrates perfumery practice with the chemical behavior of plant-based ingredients. Unlike conventional perfumers, natural perfumers work with complex, natural substances that vary by species, harvest, and origin, requiring adaptability and informed formulation choices.

In this chapter, you will explore how to select the right essential oils to mirror popular scent profiles, how to substitute synthetic notes with natural counterparts, and how to assess the quality of essential oils to ensure consistency in your perfume clones.

This is where the blend is developed through deliberate material selection and proportion.

Reconstructing the Scent with Essential Oils

The next step is to attempt the reconstruction using your existing stock of essential oils. Some aspects of commercial perfumes cannot be matched exactly with essential oils alone. However, a recognizable result can be achieved through careful material selection and skilled blending.

Begin with the base structure. Since these notes take the longest to develop and bind the whole composition, building upward from the base often yields better structural stability. For instance, if the base of the target fragrance includes sandalwood, labdanum, and patchouli, you might start by mixing small proportions of each and evaluating the result. From there, layer in the heart notes—perhaps a blend of rose, geranium, and ylang ylang—adjusting proportion as needed. Finally, add your top notes such as bergamot, petitgrain, or grapefruit, giving the clone a sparkling, fresh opening.

Throughout the process, you may find that certain essential oils offer overlapping aromatic qualities. Lavender can lend both top and heart note nuances. Frankincense may read as both fresh and resinous. Use these multifaceted oils strategically to support your blend and round off any sharp edges.

Dilution is key. Always blend your formula in a small trial quantity (1–2 mL) diluted in alcohol or a suitable carrier, so the materials can bloom and evolve as they would in a finished perfume. Allow the blend to rest for at least 24–48 hours before evaluating again.

Balancing and Refining the Clone Over Time

Cloning a fragrance is rarely a one-step operation. It is an iterative process: you start with an initial structure and refine proportion and balance over time. As your clone ages and matures, certain notes may become more prominent or fade. Take careful notes during each evaluation and adjust your formula accordingly.

If the citrus top notes are too fleeting, consider adding a more persistent supporting note, such as litsea cubeba or lemongrass. If the floral heart feels too dense, introduce a bright counterpoint, such as neroli or coriander seed. If the base is too dark or heavy, a hint of vanilla CO_2 or a lighter wood like hinoki may bring it into balance.

Over time, cloning practice often leads to original variation as structural understanding improves. This book, however, focuses on reconstruction and controlled adjustment for alignment with an original fragrance.

Selecting Essential Oils to Match Popular Scent Profiles

Designer perfumes often contain abstract accords crafted from synthetic molecules. Cloning these fragrances using only essential oils and natural extracts means identifying and matching those aroma characteristics with plant-based materials.

Step 1: Break Down the Target Perfume

Use your deconstruction process from earlier chapters to determine:

- Top notes (e.g., citrus, herbs)
- Heart notes (e.g., floral, fruity, green)
- Base notes (e.g., woods, resins, musk)

Step 2: Identify Natural Counterparts

Here are some examples of how to match essential oils to familiar perfume elements:

Scent Profile	Natural Essential Oil Matches
Sparkling citrus	Bergamot, Sweet Orange, Lemon, Grapefruit
Fresh herbal	Basil, Lavender, Rosemary, Sage
Green/crisp	Galbanum, Petitgrain, Violet Leaf
Powdery floral	Rose, Violet Absolute, Orris Root (tincture or butter)
Sensual floral	Jasmine Absolute, Ylang Ylang, Tuberose
Warm spice	Clove, Cinnamon, Cardamom, Nutmeg
Sweet gourmand	Vanilla Oleoresin, Benzoin, Cocoa Absolute
Woody depth	Cedarwood, Sandalwood, Vetiver
Resinous/ambery	Labdanum, Myrrh, Frankincense, Styrax

Scent Profile	Natural Essential Oil Matches
Earthy/mossy	Patchouli, Oakmoss Absolute, Vetiver
Animalic / musky	Ambrette Seed, Costus Root, Civet (castoreum resinoid or fossilized amber infusions)

Step 3: Layer with Nuance

To mirror the complexity of designer scents, combine oils into accords—blends that replicate a specific olfactory effect. For example:

- A white floral accord may include jasmine, neroli, and ylang ylang.
- A leather accord might blend birch tar, styrax, and labdanum.

Matching doesn't always mean duplicating a note exactly. Often, it is about evoking the impression of a note using available botanicals.

Substituting Natural Ingredients for Synthetics

Most commercial perfumes are built on a foundation of synthetic aroma chemicals—molecules that often have no natural equivalent. These synthetics provide the stability, longevity, and consistency expected in mass-market perfumery. For natural perfumers, this presents a creative challenge: approximating the impact of synthetic notes using botanical materials.

One of the most common synthetic notes is musk, which lends warmth, sensuality, and fixative qualities to perfume. True animal musks are no longer used due to ethical and legal concerns, and modern synthetic musks are entirely lab-created. However, ambrette seed CO_2 extract or tincture, derived from Abelmoschus moschatus seeds, provides a subtle, plant-based musky note with gentle floral undertones.

Another synthetic effect often found in modern perfumes is "ozone," a note designed to evoke air, water, and open space. While no natural material smells exactly like ozone, a similar airy freshness can be achieved with essential oils like violet leaf absolute, eucalyptus, or even a light touch of peppermint. Aldehydic lift—common in fragrances such as Chanel No. 5—can be approximated using high-citral essential oils such as litsea cubeba or lemongrass.

In gourmand perfumes, synthetic vanilla (vanillin or ethyl vanillin) creates sweet, creamy notes. Natural alternatives include vanilla absolute, benzoin resin, and tonka bean absolute, which together can recreate the warmth and sweetness found in many dessert-like perfumes.

Replacing synthetics requires an understanding not only of aroma but also of function. Many synthetic materials act as fixatives, slowing evaporation and supporting fragrance structure. In natural formulations, this role is often fulfilled by heavier base materials, which help anchor more volatile notes.

Here are a few common synthetic notes and their natural substitutes:

Synthetic Scent	Natural Alternative
Aldehydic effect	Lemongrass, Litsea Cubeba
Marine/Oceanic	Seaweed Absolute, Coriander Seed, Vetiver with a touch of mint
Ozonic	Violet Leaf Absolute, Eucalyptus, or Green Galbanum
Vanilla (synthetic vanillin)	Vanilla Absolute, Benzoin, Peru Balsam
Musk	Ambrette Seed CO_2 or tincture, Angelica Root, Labdanum

Tip: Don't try to mimic every synthetic precisely. Instead, focus on capturing the fragrance's overall impression and character.

Decoding the Original Scent Profile

To mirror the structure of a designer fragrance, begin by identifying its dominant notes and overall character. This information is often available through fragrance databases, reviews, and olfactory breakdowns shared by perfume enthusiasts. For example, a fragrance such as Yves Saint Laurent's *Black Opium* is commonly described as featuring vanilla and coffee wrapped in white florals, resting on a warm amber–patchouli base.

Once the fragrance has been deconstructed, you can begin selecting essential oils that express similar olfactory qualities. This involves identifying the top, middle, and base notes, as well as the overall fragrance family—floral, amber (oriental), woody, fresh, chypre, fougère, or gourmand.

It is important to understand that essential oils are inherently complex. Unlike synthetic aroma chemicals, which are designed to deliver precise, isolated scent impressions, natural materials often express multiple facets at once. As a result, a natural clone may present as richer, softer, or more organic than the original. The objective is not literal duplication, but faithful interpretation.

1. Analyze the Fragrance Pyramid

Start by researching the perfume's fragrance notes you are trying to emulate. For example:

- *Chanel No. 5* features aldehydic top notes, a floral heart of jasmine and rose, and a warm base of sandalwood and vetiver.
- *Dior Sauvage* features spicy bergamot and pepper top notes, a lavender and patchouli heart, and a base built around ambroxan, offering dry, ambergris-like diffusion.

Once you have broken down the fragrance, choose essential oils that offer similar aromatic qualities. Here are some examples:

Designer Note	Natural Material Used for Approximation
Bergamot	Bergamot (*Citrus bergamia*)
Jasmine	Jasmine Absolute (*Jasminum grandiflorum*)
Amber (Oriental)	Benzoin (*Styrax tonkinensis*) or Labdanum
Musk	Ambrette Seed CO_2 extract or tincture (*Abelmoschus moschatus*)
Sandalwood	Sandalwood (*Santalum album*) or amyris (budget option)

Essential oils often need to be layered to replicate the complexity of a synthetic perfume note. For instance, mimicking "leather" might involve a blend of birch tar, patchouli, and labdanum. A creamy "vanilla" note could be achieved using benzoin, vanilla CO_2, and a touch of tonka bean absolute.

2. Familiarize Yourself with Fragrance Families

Knowing which oils belong to which scent family supports informed material selection. For example:

- **Florals**: rose, ylang ylang, neroli, jasmine, lavender
- **Woody**: cedarwood, sandalwood, vetiver, amyris
- **Amber (Oriental)**: patchouli, myrrh, frankincense, vanilla
- **Fresh/Citrus**: lemon, lime, grapefruit, petitgrain, orange

Understanding Variations in Essential Oil Quality

Successful perfume cloning depends not only on choosing the right materials but on selecting versions of those materials that best align with the structural role they are intended to play. When working with natural materials, consistency can be elusive. Unlike synthetic molecules, essential oils vary greatly from batch to batch. Their aroma can be influenced by climate, soil, altitude, harvest time, and extraction methods. These variations affect not only the scent but also the performance and harmony of the finished fragrance.

For example, lavender grown at high altitudes in France tends to produce a sweeter, more floral aroma with typically higher proportions of linalyl acetate. In contrast, lavender from Bulgaria may have a more herbal, camphorous quality. These differences matter, especially when you are trying to match a specific scent profile.

Extraction methods also influence the quality of essential oils. Steam distillation, solvent extraction, and CO_2 extraction can yield vastly different aromatic outcomes from the same plant material. Jasmine absolute, extracted with solvents, has a richer, more indolic scent than any steam-distilled alternative. Similarly, CO_2-extracted oils often retain a fuller, more complete profile of the original plant and are especially useful for mimicking complex or deep notes.

Quality is also affected by adulteration—a common issue in the essential oil industry. Some oils are diluted with cheaper substitutes or even mixed with synthetic fragrance components. This not only undermines your efforts to stay natural but also compromises the scent and structural reliability of your formulation. To avoid this, always purchase oils from reputable suppliers that provide third-party GC/MS (gas chromatography/mass spectrometry) analysis to confirm purity and botanical origin.

Finally, aging plays a role in how certain essential oils perform in perfumery. Oils like patchouli, vetiver, and sandalwood deepen and mellow over time, making them more suitable for base notes. Conversely, citrus oils oxidize quickly and lose their sparkle, making freshness and proper storage essential.

Practical Guidance for Cloning with Natural Materials

- **Create Accords**: Many synthetic notes are abstract. Combine several natural materials to mimic a fantasy scent (e.g., gardenia = tuberose + jasmine + ylang + coconut).
- **Use Tinctures & Infusions**: DIY tinctures (e.g., coffee beans, resins) or infused botanicals can add nuance unavailable in essential oils.
- **Adjust by Proportion, Not Additions:** When a clone feels off, reduce or rebalance existing materials before adding new ones.

Cloning perfumes with natural materials is an exercise in discernment rather than duplication. While an exact molecular match is not possible, a thoughtfully constructed natural perfume can echo the essence of the original fragrance while offering greater depth and warmth.

Choosing the right essential oils requires patience, practice, and an intimate familiarity with your materials. With each formulation, you refine your ability to translate commercial perfume structures into natural expressions that are both recognizable and structurally distinct.

Complete Clone Walkthrough

The following walkthrough demonstrates how the analytical methods discussed throughout this book translate into a practical reconstruction process. Rather than attempting perfect duplication on the first attempt, the goal is to illustrate how a natural perfumer moves from observation to formulation through structured analysis, material selection, and iterative refinement.

For this example, we will continue using **Estée Lauder's** *Youth-Dew*, a classic oriental-spicy fragrance known for its rich balsamic base, strong spice heart, and citrus opening.

Initial Smell Evaluation

Begin by evaluating the original perfume without attempting to identify specific ingredients. The objective is to understand the fragrance's overall character, density, and weight.

Apply *Youth-Dew* to a fragrance blotter strip and allow the alcohol to evaporate briefly before smelling.

Initial observations may include:

- A warm, spicy opening
- Noticeable citrus brightness with a sharp lift
- Rapid emergence of clove-like spice
- A dense, resinous drydown with vanilla sweetness

At this stage, the focus is not on ingredient identification but overall behavior. The perfume immediately suggests a **rich oriental structure dominated by a substantial heart and a warm, persistent base.**

Pyramid Interpretation

Next, observe how the fragrance evolves. Evaluate the scent at several intervals.

0–10 minutes (Opening)

Citrus brightness appears first, supported by a slightly sharp aldehydic lift and an early hint of spice.

10–30 minutes (Heart Development)

The fragrance quickly becomes warmer and denser. Clove-like spice and cinnamon warmth become dominant, supported by subtle floral richness.

1–3 hours (Drydown)

The drydown reveals a rich balsamic base with resinous sweetness, patchouli depth, and lingering warmth.

From these observations, the fragrance pyramid can be summarized as follows:

Top

Citrus brightness with aldehydic-style lift

Heart

Dense floral-spice core dominated by clove and cinnamon

Base

Heavy balsamic foundation of resins, vanilla warmth, and patchouli depth

Structural Analysis

Once the scent pyramid has been observed, determine the relative emphasis of each phase.

Youth-Dew is largely **base-supported**, meaning the drydown carries much of the fragrance's identity and persistence. The heart is also substantial, while the top functions mainly as an introduction to the richer core.

A practical structural estimate might appear as:

Top: approximately **25–30%**

Heart: approximately **45–50%**

Base: approximately **20–25%**

These proportions provide a structural target for the first reconstruction attempt.

Material Selection

With the fragrance structure understood, the next step is selecting natural materials that can recreate similar effects in each layer of the composition.

Top Materials

To recreate the citrus opening and slight aldehydic brightness:

- bergamot
- sweet orange
- litsea cubeba

Litsea cubeba contributes a sharp citrus brightness that can approximate the sparkling lift often produced by aldehydes in commercial perfumes.

Heart Materials

The defining character of *Youth-Dew* lies at the heart of the fragrance, where spice and floral richness combine to form its core identity.

- clove bud
- cinnamon leaf
- cardamom
- jasmine absolute
- ylang ylang

Clove and cinnamon contribute the dominant spice character, while jasmine and ylang ylang add warmth and depth that support the transition into the balsamic base.

Base Materials

The base of *Youth-Dew* is dense and persistent, relying on resinous and woody materials that anchor the composition.

- patchouli
- labdanum
- benzoin
- frankincense
- vanilla absolute

These materials create the balsamic warmth and lingering depth that define the fragrance's drydown.

First Blend

Using the structural proportions identified earlier, create an initial reconstruction blend that reflects the fragrance's observed emphasis.

The following example represents a **first structural reconstruction based on the dominant materials identified during evaluation.** Using the structural emphasis identified during analysis—approximately 25% top, 50% heart, and 25% base—the following example converts those proportions into a 100-drop experimental blend.

Citrus Lift Accord (Top)

Material	Drops	Percentage
Bergamot	10	10%
Sweet Orange	8	8%
Litsea Cubeba	7	7%
Total	25	25%

Spice Floral Core Accord (Heart)

Material	Drops	Percentage
Clove Bud	10	10%
Cinnamon Leaf	8	8%
Cardamom	8	8%
Jasmine Absolute	12	12%
Ylang Ylang	12	12%
Total	50	50%

Balsamic Resin Accord (Base)

Material	Drops	Percentage
Patchouli	8	8%
Labdanum	6	6%
Benzoin	5	5%
Frankincense	3	3%
Vanilla Absolute	3	3%
Total	25	25%

Total Blend: 100 drops

This blend serves as an initial structural reconstruction rather than a finished clone. Its purpose is to approximate the balance between citrus brightness, spice density, and balsamic depth observed in the original fragrance.

Allow the blend to rest for **24–48 hours** before evaluation.

Evaluation

Evaluate the reconstruction alongside the original perfume using separate fragrance blotter strips.

Observe both scents at several intervals:

Opening **(0–10 minutes)**

Heart development **(10–30 minutes)**

Early drydown **(30–120 minutes)**

Extended drydown **(2–6 hours)**

During evaluation, consider the following questions:

Does the opening deliver comparable brightness and lift?

Is the spice character in the heart sufficiently dense?

Does the base provide appropriate warmth and persistence?

The first blend rarely matches the original exactly, but it should reproduce the fragrance's overall balance and progression.

Adjustment

Most perfume reconstructions require several rounds of refinement.

- **If the opening appears dull** compared to the original fragrance, increase citrus brightness slightly or reinforce the litsea cubeba component.
- **If the heart lacks body**, increase clove or cinnamon slightly while maintaining floral support.
- **If the base fades too quickly**, reinforce the composition with additional patchouli, benzoin, or labdanum.

Adjust only one or two materials at a time, allowing each revision to rest before re-evaluating. Through repeated evaluation and adjustment, the reconstruction gradually approaches the recognizable character of the original perfume.

Purpose of the Walkthrough

This walkthrough demonstrates how perfume cloning functions as a structured analytical process rather than guesswork. By observing how a fragrance behaves over time and translating those observations into material selection and proportion, the perfumer gains insight into how complex perfumes are constructed.

With continued practice, this method strengthens the ability to recognize fragrance balance, anticipate material interactions, and recreate recognizable scent profiles using natural aromatic materials.

CHAPTER 7
Natural Material Approximation

In fragrance cloning, working exclusively with natural materials introduces additional constraints that affect accuracy, longevity, and diffusion. Many commercial perfumes rely on synthetic aroma chemicals to achieve precision, projection, and stability that cannot be replicated exactly with botanically derived materials alone. This chapter illustrates how natural material approximation functions within those limits and clarifies what can and cannot reasonably be achieved.

The examples presented here are intended to demonstrate **structural reasoning**, not to provide definitive formulas or guarantee equivalence to the original fragrance.

The Role of Approximation in Natural Cloning

When cloning with naturals only, the objective shifts from duplication to **functional resemblance**. Natural materials often have broader aromatic profiles, greater batch variability, and shorter longevity than their synthetic counterparts. As a result, approximation focuses on preserving:

- Overall balance and weight
- Direction of development from opening to drydown
- Relative emphasis of structural layers
- Recognizable character of the original fragrance

Exact replication of aroma intensity, sharpness, or projection should not be expected.

Example: Natural Approximation of an Oriental-Spicy Structure

Amber (Oriental)-spicy perfumes often rely heavily on synthetics for warmth, diffusion, and longevity. When approximating such a structure using natural materials, the emphasis must be placed on **layered density and fixation**.

A natural material approach may include:

- **Opening:** Citrus oils combined with lightly aromatic or herbaceous materials to introduce brightness without excessive volatility
- **Heart:** Warm spices and florals selected for persistence and body rather than sharpness
- **Base:** Balsams, resins, woods, and roots chosen to provide depth, continuity, and anchoring

In this context, the base structure becomes especially critical, as natural materials typically evaporate more quickly and require additional support to maintain presence.

Addressing the Absence of Synthetic Effects

Certain effects common in commercial perfumery—such as intense aldehydic lift, clean musky diffusion, or extreme longevity—are difficult to reproduce naturally. When these effects are central to a fragrance's identity, natural approximation requires strategic compromise.

Approaches may include:

- **Replacing sharp synthetic** lift with softer radiance through citrus, aromatic herbs, or light resins
- **Building perceived warmth** through layered balsams rather than amber chemicals
- **Accepting reduced projection** in favor of structural coherence

The success of a natural approximation should be measured by **recognizability**, not parity.

Evaluating Natural Approximations

Evaluation of natural clones follows the same comparative process outlined earlier in this book, but should be interpreted with adjusted expectations. Key questions include:

Does the fragrance align with the same family and recognizable character as the reference?
Does the structure develop in a similar sequence, even if more softly?
Does the base support the fragrance long enough to preserve identity?

Discrepancies should be addressed structurally—by reinforcing layers or adjusting proportions—rather than by attempting to force natural materials into roles they cannot sustain.

Chapter 8

Blending Techniques for Fragrance Cloning

In natural perfumery—and especially in fragrance cloning— how you structure and layer essential oils will determine whether your creation evokes the same emotional and olfactory experience as the original. This chapter outlines multiple blending strategies: by note, by accord, by aromatic group, and for performance factors such as longevity and sillage. For each method, we'll include clear, practical steps so you can confidently apply them in your perfume cloning process.

Blending by Note

In fragrance cloning, blending by note is a method of structural reconstruction rather than creative composition. The purpose is not to define top, heart, and base notes, but to identify how the inspiration fragrance is weighted across its evaporation curve and to replicate that distribution in your formula.

Every commercial perfume emphasizes one or more stages of its development. Some perfumes emphasize the opening, others the heart, while many derive their signature from the drydown. Successful cloning begins with observing where the fragrance carries its greatest impact and designing the blend to reflect that same temporal balance.

When building a clone, the formulation should be constructed in reverse order—base to heart to top—to allow the heavier materials to establish a stable foundation before lighter notes are introduced. This approach supports smoother integration and provides greater control over how the fragrance unfolds over time.

Rather than attempting to match individual notes exactly, the goal is to mirror the original perfume's progression: its opening, development, and drydown. When the structural emphasis is accurate, the resulting clone will feel familiar and recognizable, even when working exclusively with natural materials.

How to Blend by Note

1. **Analyze the Note Emphasis of the Original Fragrance**

   Begin by evaluating how the inspiration perfume behaves over time. Determine whether its character is most prominent in the opening, the heart, or the drydown. This assessment—not predefined oil categories—should guide how you assign materials to the top, heart, and base structure of your clone.

2. Select Materials Based on Functional Role

Choose essential oils based on their role in the original fragrance, not just by name. Identify which materials in your palette can replicate brightness, diffusion, body, or depth. In cloning, materials are chosen for how they behave within the structure, not simply where they traditionally sit in the pyramid.

3. Establish a Structural Ratio that Mirrors the Original

Use the olfactory balance of the inspiration fragrance to guide your proportions. A balanced composition may resemble a traditional distribution. At the same time, a fresh or fleeting perfume may require a stronger top structure, and a deep or resinous fragrance may demand greater weight in the base. Ratios should reflect the original's perceived emphasis rather than follow a fixed formula.

4. Build the Formula from Base to Top

Construct the blend in reverse order: start with the base materials, then the heart, and finish with the top structure. This approach allows heavier components to integrate fully before lighter materials are introduced, resulting in a more cohesive and controllable reconstruction.

5. Evaluate Integration and Adjust Structurally

Blend in small test batches and allow the formula to rest before evaluation. When assessing the blend, focus on whether the emphasis matches the original fragrance—whether the opening feels too sharp or too weak, the heart lacks presence, or the base does not anchor the composition adequately. Adjust by reinforcing or reducing entire layers rather than chasing individual notes.

Successful blending by note begins with identifying the dominant stage of the reference perfume. When the structural emphasis is correct, the clone will feel recognizable even if individual ingredients differ.

Blending by Accord: Structural Frameworks in Fragrance Cloning

Most commercial perfumes are not built material by material, but around recognizable accord frameworks that give the fragrance its identity. Identifying and reconstructing these frameworks is often the most efficient way to reproduce a perfume's character using natural materials.

In cloning, an accord is treated as a unified olfactory structure rather than a collection of individual materials. Accords are used to replicate familiar perfume families and signature structures commonly found in designer fragrances. Common accord frameworks frequently encountered in commercial perfumery are summarized in the reference chart later in the resource section.

Understanding how these accords function allows the natural perfumer to reconstruct the backbone of many commercial perfumes, even when the exact formula is unknown.

When reconstructing a fragrance, accords can be built in two primary ways, depending on the original perfume's structure.

Horizontal Accords

Horizontal accords are constructed within a single layer of the fragrance pyramid. They are used to strengthen or replicate a specific phase of the perfume's development. For example, a citrus opening may rely on a horizontal top accord composed of multiple citrus materials, while a floral heart may be built from several complementary floral oils. Horizontal accords are most useful when a particular stage of the fragrance stands out strongly in the original perfume.

Vertical Accords

Vertical accords, by contrast, span the top, heart, and base simultaneously. These accords form a complete, self-contained scent structure and are often responsible for a perfume's overall signature. In cloning, vertical accords are particularly valuable when the original fragrance presents as cohesive and unified rather than sharply layered. A gourmand vertical accord, for example, may combine a bright opening, a floral or creamy heart, and a sweet, persistent base to reproduce the perfume's core identity in a single construction.

How to Blend by Accord: Reproducing Recognizable Perfume Signatures

When cloning a perfume, blending by accord begins with identifying which type of structure best replicates the original fragrance. If the inspiration perfume places strong emphasis on a specific stage—such as a distinctive citrus opening or a pronounced floral heart—a horizontal accord is most appropriate. Horizontal accords are used to reconstruct individual layers of the fragrance pyramid. When the goal is to reproduce a perfume's overall theme or signature, a vertical accord is often more effective. Vertical accords combine materials from the top, heart, and base to define the fragrance's core structure.

Once the accord type is selected, construct the accord using three to five essential oils. In horizontal accords, one material typically serves as the dominant note, supported by one or two secondary materials and, if needed, a subtle enhancer. A useful starting proportion is approximately 40% dominant material, 30% supporting material, 20% modifying material, and 10% enhancer. For vertical accords, a balanced structure often follows a ratio of roughly 30% top notes, 40% heart notes, and 30% base notes, adjusted as needed to reflect the inspiration fragrance's style and emphasis.

Before incorporating an accord into a full perfume formula, test it independently. Blend a small batch—usually 5 to 10 total drops—and allow it to rest for 1 to 2 days so the materials can integrate. Evaluate the accord by comparing it directly to the inspiration fragrance, focusing on whether it captures the same character, weight, and progression rather than on individual notes.

Once refined, the accord can be incorporated into a complete perfume composition. A vertical amber accord, for example, may serve as the structural foundation of a clone, with additional top and heart materials added to complete the reconstruction. In this way, accords function as modular building blocks, allowing you to replicate commercial fragrance structures with precision rather than assembling blends oil by oil without a clear architectural framework.

How to Blend by Accord (Cloning Method)

1. Identify the Dominant Structural Accord

Evaluate the inspiration fragrance to determine whether its identity is driven by a recognizable accord framework, such as amber, fougère, chypre, gourmand, or floral bouquet. This assessment should focus on the overall structural impression rather than isolated notes.

2. Determine the Accord Orientation

Decide whether the fragrance is best represented by a horizontal accord, emphasizing a specific stage of the fragrance pyramid, or a vertical accord that spans the top, heart, and base simultaneously. This choice should reflect how the perfume presents as it develops on the skin.

3. Select Core Materials for the Accord

Choose three to five essential oils that collectively reproduce the character of the identified accord. One material should serve as the dominant anchor of the accord, supported by secondary materials that contribute body, texture, or nuance.

4. Establish Internal Accord Balance

Adjust the proportions within the accord to reflect the weight and emphasis of the original fragrance. Horizontal accords should reinforce the targeted stage of development, while vertical accords should maintain balance across volatility levels to form a cohesive structure.

5. **Evaluate the Accord Independently**

   Test the accord on its own before incorporating it into a full perfume formula. Allow it to rest, then assess whether it captures the character, density, and progression of the inspiration fragrance at a structural level rather than by individual note accuracy.

6. **Integrate the Accord into the Full Composition**

   Once refined, incorporate the accord into the broader perfume structure, using it as a foundational building block. Additional materials may be layered around the accord to complete the reconstruction while preserving the accord's role as the core framework of the clone.

Blending by Aromatic Group

Blending by aromatic group is most effective in fragrance cloning when the exact note pyramid or accord structure of the original perfume cannot be clearly identified. In these cases, the fragrance can often still be understood—and reconstructed—by recognizing its dominant aromatic family. Many commercial perfumes communicate their identity through an overall aromatic character rather than through easily distinguishable individual notes.

.By identifying the primary aromatic group a fragrance belongs to, the natural perfumer can recreate its general structure and recognizable character even in the absence of detailed formulation data. This method functions as a diagnostic shortcut, allowing you to approximate the perfume's framework before refining it through note emphasis or accord reconstruction.

Common aromatic groups used in perfumery include:

- **Citrus:** Bright, uplifting, and fresh (lemon, orange, grapefruit)
- **Floral:** Romantic, classic, and expressive (rose, jasmine, ylang ylang)
- **Woody:** Dry, grounding, and structural (cedarwood, vetiver, sandalwood)
- **Spicy:** Warm, energizing, and dynamic (clove, cardamom, black pepper)
- **Green:** Crisp, leafy, and fresh (galbanum, violet leaf)
- **Gourmand:** Sweet, edible, and comforting (vanilla, cocoa, tonka)

When cloning a fragrance using this approach, begin by determining which aromatic group dominates the perfume's overall impression. The goal is not to catalog individual notes, but to identify the family that defines how the fragrance reads as a whole. Secondary groups are then used strategically to modify, balance, or support the dominant character.

A practical reconstruction strategy is to establish the core of the blend using materials from the dominant aromatic group, introduce a complementary group in a supporting role to provide contrast or lift, and anchor the composition with a base material that stabilizes the structure. This approach allows you to recreate a fragrance's recognizable identity while maintaining structural accuracy.

How to Blend by Aromatic Group (Cloning Method)

1. **Identify the Dominant Aromatic Group**

   Evaluate the fragrance as a whole and determine which aromatic family defines its primary character. This assessment should be based on the overall impression rather than isolated notes.

2. **Establish the Core Structure**

   Select two materials from the dominant aromatic group to form the foundation of the reconstruction and clearly establish the perfume's identity.

3. **Introduce a Complementary Modifier**

   Add one material from a complementary aromatic group to adjust balance, contrast, or diffusion without altering the primary character. The modifier should enhance the dominant group rather than compete with it.

4. **Anchor the Composition**

   Incorporate one anchoring material—typically a wood, resin, balsam, or other low-volatility component—to provide stability and support the fragrance's evolution over time.

When evaluating the blend, assess whether the dominant aromatic group remains clearly recognizable and whether the overall structure aligns with the character of the inspiration fragrance. Adjustments should be made at the structural level rather than by chasing individual note accuracy.

Example: Aromatic Group Reconstruction

If cloning a fragrance that presents as a soft gourmand floral, begin by establishing the gourmand core using materials such as vanilla and tonka. Introduce a floral modifier—such as jasmine—to refine the sweetness and add dimension without shifting the dominant character. Anchor the composition with a stabilizing base material, such as benzoin or sandalwood, to support longevity and cohesion.

In this structure, the gourmand materials define the fragrance identity, the floral modifier provides balance and lift, and the anchoring material ensures structural stability.

Common Aromatic Group Frameworks

Accord Type	Example Oils	Note
Amber	Labdanum, Vanilla, Benzoin, Tonka, Peru Balsam, Styrax, Myrrh, Opoponax	Base
Chypre	Bergamot, Patchouli, Labdanum, Oakmoss Absolute	Base
Fougère	Lavender, Geranium, Tonka	Heart
Citrus	Lemon, Bergamot, Grapefruit	Top
Floral	Rose, Ylang Ylang, Jasmine	Heart
Leather	Birch Tar, Labdanum, Clove	Base
Green	Galbanum, Violet Leaf, Basil	Heart

These frameworks serve as reference structures to support the identification and reconstruction of aromatic groups. They are not fixed formulas and should be adjusted to reflect the fragrance being cloned's style and balance.

Blending for Longevity and Sillage

In fragrance cloning, accuracy is measured not only by scent resemblance but also by performance. A successful clone must approximate the original perfume's longevity and projection, which are determined primarily by structural formulation choices rather than application techniques.

Longevity is governed by the proportion and placement of low-volatility materials within the formula. Clones that fade too quickly often lack sufficient base structure or rely too heavily on volatile top materials. To increase longevity, the formula should incorporate stable fixative materials—such as labdanum, patchouli, vetiver, benzoin, or other resinous components—and ensure the base structure carries enough weight to support the composition over time.

Sillage, or scent projection, is influenced by how effectively volatile and semi-volatile materials are balanced within the blend. Bright, diffusive materials—particularly citrus, aromatic herbs, or lightly camphoraceous oils—contribute lift and initial projection, while well-chosen bridging materials help connect the opening to the heart without causing sharpness or imbalance. Excessive volatility without structural support may increase projection briefly but will compromise longevity and cohesion.

When evaluating cloning performance, assess the formula as a whole rather than focusing on individual materials. Compare the clone and the inspiration fragrance side by side over several hours, noting differences in projection, persistence, and dry-down presence. Adjustments should be made structurally—by reinforcing or reducing entire layers or functional roles—rather than by adding isolated "boosting" ingredients.

Matching performance is ultimately a matter of architectural balance. When the structural framework is correct, longevity and sillage will emerge naturally as properties of the formula rather than requiring corrective techniques.

CHAPTER 9

From Analysis to Reconstruction

Fragrance cloning is a structured process that involves analyzing an existing perfume, identifying its aromatic components and structural relationships, and reconstructing those elements using essential oils and other natural materials. Rather than focusing on novelty, this approach emphasizes careful observation, proportion, and material behavior. For natural perfumers, cloning is a technical discipline that develops sensory discrimination and formulation skills through deliberate reconstruction.

Instructions for Making a Clone Perfume

Materials Needed:

- Original perfume (the one you want to replicate)
- Essential oils or absolutes (similar to those in the original perfume)
- Carrier oil (such as jojoba) or perfumer's alcohol

- Glass droppers or pipettes
- Amber glass bottles
- Scent strips
- Notebook or perfumer's journal for recording formulations
- Digital scale capable of measuring to 0.01 g

Steps:

1. Analyze the Original Fragrance:
   a) Spray the original fragrance: Spritz the perfume onto a scent strip or blotter paper.
   b) Observe and Document: Carefully smell the fragrance at different intervals (immediately, after 15 minutes, and after an hour) to identify dominance shifts and structural development over time. Take detailed notes on your observations.

2. Research the Original Fragrance:
   a) Consult published note breakdowns and community analyses in perfume databases to confirm structural emphasis, accords, and performance observations.

3. Select Your Ingredients:
   a) Based on your analysis and research, choose essential oils and absolutes that match the identified notes of the original fragrance.

4. Create a Basic Formula:
   a) Start Simple: Begin with a simple formula that includes a few drops of each of the identified top, middle, and base

notes. For example, a ratio of 30% top notes, 50% middle notes, and 20% base notes is an exploratory starting point only.

b) Record Everything: Write down the exact number of drops or weight of each ingredient you use.

5. Blend and Test:

a) Combine the Ingredients: In a small amber glass bottle, combine your selected ingredients. If using a carrier oil, fill the bottle about 90% full and add the essential oils to the remaining 10%. For an alcohol base, mix the essential oils first and then add the alcohol.

b) Shake and Rest: Shake the bottle gently to mix the ingredients. Let the blend rest for a few days to allow the scents to meld together.

6. Evaluate and Adjust:

a) Test the Blend: Apply a small amount of the blend to a scent strip or your skin and compare it to the original perfume.

b) Adjust as Needed: If the clone perfume doesn't match closely enough, adjust the formula by adjusting proportions or structural emphasis. Record each adjustment meticulously.

7. Age the Perfume:

a) Let it Mature: Once you're satisfied with the blend, let the perfume age for at least a few weeks. This allows the scents to develop and integrate fully.

8. Final Testing:

a) Compare Again: After aging, test the perfume again against the original. Make any final adjustments if necessary.

b) Final Blend: Once you're satisfied, scale up the formula to make a larger batch while maintaining the same proportions.

9. Bottle and Label:

a) Store Properly: Transfer the finished perfume to a clean amber glass bottle for storage. Amber bottles help protect the perfume from light degradation.

b) Label Your Creation: Clearly label the bottle with the perfume name and the date it was created.

Making Your Own Signature Scent from a Clone

A natural progression of the cloning process is to arrive at a fragrance that is truly your own—an expression of taste, personality, and mood. This signature scent can evolve over time, just as you do.

To craft your signature scent:

1. **Start with your best clone** – the one that is closest to a fragrance you already love.

2. **Tweak based on your feedback** – note where the clone differs from your expectations and begin adjusting.

3. **Incorporate your favorite notes** – even if they weren't in the original formula, they can make the fragrance yours.

4. **Simplify if needed** – sometimes a signature scent emerges from paring down complexity. A clean, minimal blend of just three or four beautifully balanced oils can be just as powerful as a complex formula.

5. **Name your blend** – giving your scent a name makes it feel personal and official. It marks the moment when your fragrance becomes uniquely yours.

Remember, perfume is as much an emotional experience as it is a chemical one. Your signature blend should evoke feelings, memories, and a sense of identity. Cloning may start with reconstruction, but customization is where artistry begins.

Experimenting with New Notes and Accords

Use the clone as a structural base and introduce one new note or accord at a time to observe how the composition shifts. Document each iteration carefully, including drop counts, percentages, and evaluation notes, to ensure reproducibility and informed comparison.

Approaches to experimentation include introducing controlled contrast—such as adding a small amount of green galbanum to lift a floral structure or a measured spice like cardamom to add warmth to a woody framework. You may also develop structured variations that emphasize different use contexts by adjusting weight or diffusion, such as a softer daytime version or a denser evening interpretation.

When unsure of direction, preliminary layering tests with single materials or reference blends can help identify promising adjustments before committing to the formula. This allows exploration without destabilizing the core structure.

Development Process for the Clone

The following natural clone was developed using essential oils to recreate the character and structural behavior of *Chanel No. 5*, a classic floral-aldehydic perfume. Working with natural materials requires analytical judgment, estimation, and creative decision-making. The steps below outline the process used to develop this clone and can be applied to other fragrances throughout your own cloning work.

Step 1: Identify the Target Fragrance's Structure

Begin by researching the fragrance and gathering publicly available information such as the note breakdown (top, middle, and base), fragrance family, and key accords or impressions, including qualities like powdery, soapy, floral, or creamy.

In this example, the original fragrance is a classic floral aldehydic composition characterized by prominent synthetic aldehydes, ylang ylang, rose, jasmine, sandalwood, vetiver, vanilla, and a powdery musk base. Because this reconstruction uses only essential oils, those synthetic effects are translated into natural materials that create a similar overall impression.

Step 2: Choose Natural Substitutes for Key Effects

This step relies on an understanding of how essential oils behave and function within a fragrance structure.

- **Aldehydic effects (synthetic):** The sparkling, fizzy, and soapy lift of synthetic aldehydes can be approximated using bright citrus oils such as litsea cubeba, lemon, and bergamot.
- **Jasmine and Rose:** Jasmine absolute and rose otto form the primary floral heart, establishing the classic richness associated with the inspiration fragrance.
- **Ylang Ylang:** Ylang Ylang contributes creamy, rounded floral notes with a subtle banana-like nuance, enhancing softness and cohesion.
- **Base structure:** Sandalwood, vetiver, patchouli, and vanilla recreate the warm, sensual foundation of the original composition using natural materials.
- **Supporting modifiers:** Geranium, clary sage, and lavender introduce green, herbal, and lightly spicy facets that add complexity and balance to the floral core.

Step 3: Estimate Drop Ratios by Note Category

Perfumes are traditionally structured according to relative note weight and evaporation rate, approximate ranges often used as a starting point—commonly 25% top notes, 45% heart notes, and 30% base notes.

For a 100-drop test blend, this structure translates to the following proportions: 25 drops to the top structure, 45 to the heart, and 30 to the base.

This distribution creates vertical balance within the clone. Heavier, longer-lasting materials are used in smaller quantities but exert greater influence over time, while lighter top notes provide brightness and initial impact before dissipating more quickly.

Step 4: Trial, Evaluation, and Adjustment

Establish initial proportions based on each material's relative strength and persistence. Potent oils, such as vetiver, should be used sparingly, while lighter materials may require higher drop counts to register clearly.

Allow the blend to rest for several days before evaluation to observe how the fragrance develops through the drydown. A composition that appears sharp or unbalanced immediately after blending may soften, integrate, or shift significantly with short-term aging.

Evaluate the blend methodically, take detailed notes, and make adjustments as needed. If the clone feels overly sweet or dense, reduce the use of heavy floral or sweet materials, such as jasmine or vanilla. If the opening lacks lift, increase bright top notes like bergamot or litsea cubeba. If the floral heart feels flat or muted, small additions of geranium can introduce freshness and clarity.

Step 5: Final Refinement and Aging

After adjusting the initial blend, allow it to age for two to four weeks, then re-evaluate its development from top to base over several hours. This extended resting period reveals how the materials integrate and how the structure evolves.

If necessary, prepare a second trial blend with small, targeted adjustments. For example, if the rose note feels too heavy, substituting rose geranium for rose otto may lighten the floral impression without compromising structure.

Developing a natural perfume clone follows a clear progression: researching the fragrance's note pyramid, family, and key accords; translating synthetic effects into essential oils; establishing top, heart, and base structure; blending and testing using informed drop ratios; and refining the formula through aging, evaluation, and adjustment.

Natural *Chanel No. 5*–Inspired Fragrance Clone

This natural version captures the floral richness, powdery depth, and elegant sparkle of *Chanel No. 5* without synthetic aldehydes or musk. Litsea cubeba acts as a natural aldehydic booster, and the balance of ylang ylang, rose, jasmine, and sandalwood brings a creamy, powdery sophistication.

Top Notes (25%)

Material	Drops	Percentage
Bergamot	10	10%
Lemon	6	6%
Petitgrain	5	5%
Litsea Cubeba	4	4%
Total	25	25%

Heart Notes (45%)

Material	Drops	Percentage
Ylang Ylang	12	12%
Rose Otto	10	10%
Jasmine Absolute	8	8%
Geranium	6	6%
Lavender	5	5%
Clary Sage	4	4%
Total	45	45%

Base Notes (30%)

Material	Drops	Percentage
Sandalwood	10	10%
Vetiver	6	6%
Vanilla Absolute or CO_2	6	6%
Frankincense	4	4%
Patchouli	4	4%
Total	30	30%

Total = 100 drops

Instructions

1. Blend the essential oils in a small glass bottle to create the aromatic concentrate.
2. Add perfumer's alcohol or carrier oil to reach the desired total volume (approximately 10 mL).
3. Shake gently to thoroughly combine the materials.
4. Allow the blend to rest for at least 72 hours. For a more accurate evaluation, let it age for 2–4 weeks to allow the structure to integrate fully.
5. Test on a blotter or skin and adjust as needed. If the blend is too floral, reduce rose or jasmine. If the powdery character is too strong, soften the base by reducing vetiver or increasing citrus in the opening.

CHAPTER 10

Testing and Perfecting Your Perfume Clone

———

Creating a perfume clone doesn't end with the first formula—and that is part of what makes the process so satisfying. Careful verification and controlled refinement transform a promising blend into a convincing reconstruction. In this chapter, you'll identify where your formula diverges from the original fragrance and make targeted adjustments to proportions and ratios through systematic testing and comparison, refining the clone's balance, character, and performance.

Evaluating Scent Development Over Time

When you first mix your clone, the scent will smell quite different from how it smells after it has rested on the skin or even in the bottle. Perfumes are dynamic; their aromas evolve as the volatile molecules evaporate at different rates. This evolution is called scent development or drydown.

Steps for evaluation:

1. **Initial Smell (Opening):** Immediately after application, the volatile materials are most noticeable. This stage typically lasts **10–30 minutes.**
2. **Heart (Development):** As the opening softens, the core character becomes clearer. This stage may last **several hours.**
3. **Base (Drydown):** The least volatile materials remain longest, shaping depth and persistence. This stage may last **several hours to a full day,** depending on the formula.

To evaluate your clone:

1. Apply a small amount to the skin or a testing strip.
2. Smell immediately, then at **15, 30, and 60 minutes,** and again over the next several hours.
3. Take notes on what is **stronger, weaker, or missing** compared to the original fragrance.
4. Note whether transitions feel **smooth and continuous** or **abrupt and uneven** relative to the reference.

Give your clone time—many formulas benefit from resting for at least 48 hours, and some continue to integrate for 1 to 2 **weeks.** Store the blend in a cool, dark place while it matures.

Adjusting Proportions and Ratios

Once you've evaluated the clone over time, you may find specific areas that need refinement. The goal is not to keep changing ingredients at random, but to adjust proportions in a controlled way until the clone converges with the reference. Common adjustments include:

- **Opening:** If the opening is too weak or fades too quickly, increase the proportion of volatile, fresh materials (e.g., citrus, aromatic herbs).
- **Heart:** If the core character is thin or indistinct, strengthen the mid-structure with longer-lasting floral, spicy, green, or aromatic materials.
- **Base:** If the drydown lacks depth or persistence, increase the proportion of base materials and fixative structure (e.g., woods, resins, musk).

Adjustment tips:

- **Make small changes**—adjust by **1–2% increments** to avoid destabilizing the structure.
- **Track every modification** using a formula sheet to compare versions accurately.
- **Work in small test batches** to conserve materials and speed iteration.
- **If a material is too harsh or dominant**, reduce it first before adding compensating ingredients.

Over time, careful iteration will align the structure. The key is consistency: change one variable at a time, evaluate again, and let the evidence guide your next move.

Refining the Clone Through Iteration

Testing and perfecting a perfume clone is an iterative process of evaluation and correction. Observing the fragrance over time reveals where the structure diverges from the reference and what needs adjustment. Fine-tuning proportions—especially at the layer or functional level—brings the formula closer to the original composition. When the structural framework is correctly balanced, longevity and projection emerge naturally as properties of the formula, and the clone becomes increasingly convincing with each controlled revision.

CHAPTER 11

Common Issues and How to Fix Them

Even the most carefully blended perfume clone can sometimes miss the mark. Whether the scent doesn't last, smells too strong, or feels "off," these issues are common and usually easy to resolve with a few adjustments. This section will guide you through the most common problems encountered in perfume cloning and offer practical solutions to fine-tune your formulation.

1. The Scent Doesn't Last (Poor Longevity)

Cause: Insufficient base notes or fixatives; high ingredient volatility.

Fix:

- Increase the concentration of base notes like vetiver, patchouli, myrrh, sandalwood, or benzoin.
- Add natural fixatives such as orris root, labdanum, or oakmoss (in safe, IFRA-compliant amounts).

- Consider using a higher essential oil concentration (move from Eau de Toilette to Eau de Parfum strength).
- Allow your blend to age (macerate) for at least 2–6 weeks before judging performance.

2. The Scent Changes Too Quickly (Unstable Drydown)

Cause: Imbalance between top, middle, and base notes.

Fix:

- Add stronger middle and base notes to anchor the top notes.
- Use essential oils with slower evaporation rates to create smoother transitions (e.g., cedarwood, frankincense, balsams).
- Blend by pyramid structure: 20% top, 50% middle, 30% base as a starting point, and adjust accordingly.

3. It Smells Too Sharp, Harsh, or Medicinal

Cause: Overuse of strong, camphoraceous or citrusy oils (e.g., eucalyptus, rosemary, tea tree).

Fix:

- Soften the formula with floral, woody, or balsamic oils, such as lavender, rose, or benzoin.
- Round out sharp edges with creamy notes such as sandalwood, vanilla CO_2, or tonka bean absolute (if using natural substitutes).

- Dilute the entire perfume with more alcohol or a carrier oil to mellow its impact.

4. It Smells Too Weak or Fades Fast on the Skin

Cause: Over-dilution, low oil concentration, or poor skin affinity.

Fix:

- Increase the percentage of essential oils (aim for 15–30% in perfume oils or extrait formulations).
- Use richer base oils for oil perfumes, such as jojoba or fractionated coconut oil, which hold scent longer.
- Apply perfume to pulse points and moisturized skin to improve longevity.

5. It Smells Too Sweet, Powdery, or Cloying

Cause: Excess of sweet or floral notes like ylang ylang, jasmine, benzoin, or vanilla.

Fix:

- Add fresh, green, or citrusy elements to cut through the heaviness (e.g., bergamot, petitgrain, basil).
- Use spices like cardamom or black pepper for contrast and balance.
- Reduce the offending note in small increments until harmony is restored.

6. The Clone Doesn't Smell Like the Original

Cause: Missing key note, inaccurate proportions, or use of substitutes.

Fix:

- Reanalyze the original perfume: identify what note might be missing (a smoky nuance? a soft floral? a musk-like warmth?).
- Compare accord by accord (top, middle, base), and evaluate which layer needs adjustment.
- Keep a testing journal and remake in small batches for comparison.
- Remember: natural-only formulas may not match synthetics perfectly, but you can still recreate the scent's feel and impression.

7. The Scent Smells Flat or Boring

Cause: Lack of contrast or complexity.

Fix:

- Add complementary contrasts: sweet vs. bitter, warm vs. cool, floral vs. resinous.
- Introduce subtle enhancers like angelica root, carrot seed, or oakwood to add intrigue.

- Experiment with layering techniques or using modifiers to bring out hidden facets of the blend.

8. Cloudiness or Sediment in Your Perfume

Cause: Incompatible oils, impurities, or lack of filtration.

Fix:

- Filter the perfume using a coffee filter or fine muslin.
- Let the perfume rest for a few weeks, then decant the clear portion.
- Some essential oils, such as resins or CO_2 extracts, may naturally cause clouding—shake before use or reformulate.

9. Skin Irritation or Sensitivity

Cause: Essential oil concentration too high or irritating oils used (e.g., cinnamon, clove, citral-rich oils).

Fix:

- Dilute to safe dermal limits (generally 1–5% for leave-on applications).
- Use a patch test and always check safety data on each essential oil used.
- Replace known irritants with gentler alternatives, such as using palmarosa instead of lemongrass.

Keep Blending Notes

Document your blends, ratios, and adjustments meticulously. Perfume creation is both science and art, and even small tweaks can make a big difference. By keeping track, you'll be able to refine your clones and become a master at troubleshooting your signature scents.

APPENDIX A
Natural Substitutes for Synthetic Notes

This chart offers natural alternatives to common synthetic fragrance notes. These substitutes aren't identical—but they can recreate a similar olfactory impression using essential oils, absolutes, CO_2 extracts, resins, and tinctures.

Fruity Notes

Synthetic Note	Natural Substitute(s)	Aroma Type
Apple	Litsea Cubeba, Galbanum, Buchu, Melissa	crisp, tart, green
Pear	Carrot Seed, Violet Leaf, Ambrette, Osmanthus	watery, soft, juicy
Strawberry	Blackcurrant Bud, Davana, Ylang Ylang, Peru Balsam	fruity, jammy, sweet

Synthetic Note	Natural Substitute(s)	Aroma Type
Peach	Osmanthus, Roman Chamomile, Mimosa, Tuberose	sweet, creamy, soft
Pineapple	Litsea Cubeba, Lemongrass, Tagetes	tropical, tangy, citrus-sweet
Mango	Tagetes, Ylang Ylang, Jasmine Sambac	exotic, ripe, floral
Passionfruit	Davana, Blackcurrant Bud, Ginger Lily	bright, exotic, tangy
Raspberry	Blackcurrant Bud, Davana, Violet Leaf	juicy, green, tart-sweet
Melon/Cucumber	Violet Leaf, Galbanum, Green Mandarin, Cucumber Tincture	fresh, dewy, aquatic-green

Gourmand Notes

Synthetic Note	Natural Substitute(s)	Aroma Type
Vanilla	Vanilla Oleoresin, Benzoin, Tolu Balsam, Tonka Bean	warm, sweet, creamy
Caramel	Benzoin, Labdanum, Tolu Balsam, Peru Balsam	burnt sugar, buttery
Cotton candy	Vanilla, Benzoin, Ylang Ylang, Cocoa Absolute	sugary, airy, candy-like

Synthetic Note	Natural Substitute(s)	Aroma Type
Chocolate	Cocoa Absolute, Coffee, Vanilla, Nutmeg	rich, bitter-sweet
Coffee	Coffee, Roasted Chicory Tincture	roasted, deep, aromatic
Honey	Beeswax Absolute, Immortelle, Mimosa, Orange Blossom	syrupy, floral-sweet
Almond/Cherry	Bitter Almond Tincture (rare), Benzoin, Tonka, Cinnamon Leaf	nutty, sweet, cherry-almond
Licorice/Aniseed	Anise, Fennel, Tarragon, Basil (methyl chavicol CT)	spicy, sweet, aromatic

Floral & Green Notes

Synthetic Note	Natural Substitute(s)	Aroma Type
Lily of the Valley	Rose, Neroli, Bergamot, Jasmine + Green Accord	fresh, clean floral
Lilac	Jasmine, Ylang Ylang, Rose Geranium, Violet Leaf	spring floral, powdery
Gardenia	Tuberose, Jasmine, Ylang Ylang + Coconut	creamy, floral, tropical

Synthetic Note	Natural Substitute(s)	Aroma Type
Hyacinth	Violet Leaf, Neroli, Orange Blossom, Green Tea Accord	green floral
Violet	Violet Leaf, Orris Root, Mimosa	powdery, soft, sweet floral
Fresh Cut Grass	Galbanum, Violet Leaf, Green Mandarin, Cucumber Tincture	sharp, green
Dewy Floral	Neroli, Violet Leaf, Green Tea Accord, Petitgrain	soft, watery floral

Wood, Resin & Earth Notes

Synthetic Note	Natural Substitute(s)	Aroma Type
Sandalwood	Santalum Album (Indian), Amyris, Copaiba, Spikenard	creamy, soft, woody
Cedar	Atlas Cedarwood, Himalayan Cedar, Virginia Cedarwood	dry, woody, pencil-shavings
Vetiver	Vetiver (aged), Patchouli, Oakmoss	earthy, smoky, green
Patchouli	Aged Patchouli, Oakmoss, Myrrh	earthy, balsamic
Incense/Smoke	Frankincense, Myrrh, Opoponax, Cade, Birch Tar	dry, smoky, resinous

Synthetic Note	Natural Substitute(s)	Aroma Type
Amber	Labdanum, Benzoin, Vanilla, Cistus	warm, sweet, resinous
Oud / Agarwood	Oud, Agarwood, Labdanum + Patchouli + Smoke Accord	woody, leather, animalic
Moss/Earth	Oakmoss, Vetiver, Patchouli, Myrrh	damp, forest-like

Fresh, Airy & Marine Notes

Synthetic Note	Natural Substitute(s)	Aroma Type
Ocean /Sea Breeze	Seaweed Absolute, Cypress, Juniper, Eucalyptus	salty, marine, fresh
Clean Linen	Lavender, Neroli, Rose Geranium, Petitgrain	soapy, floral-fresh
Metallic	Peppermint, Eucalyptus, Silver Fir, Aldehyde-like citrus	cool, bright, sharp
Rain/ozone	Eucalyptus, Galbanum, Cucumber, Spearmint, Violet Leaf	dewy, ozonic, herbal
Citrus Sparkle	Bergamot, Lemon, Lime, Grapefruit, Litsea Cubeba	bright, fresh, effervescent

Spice, Balsam & Exotic Notes

Synthetic Note	Natural Substitute(s)	Aroma Type
Cinnamon/Spice	Cinnamon Bark/ Leaf, Clove, Nutmeg, Cardamom	warm, spicy
Incense/Temple	Frankincense, Myrrh, Labdanum, Styrax	sacred, resinous
Leather	Birch Tar, Labdanum, Styrax, Cistus	smoky, animalic, dark
Tobacco	Tobacco, Vanilla, Labdanum, Cocoa	sweet, smoky, masculine
Balsamic/Sweet Resin	Benzoin, Peru Balsam, Tolu Balsam, Elemi	sweet, resinous, round

Floral Family

Floral Note	Natural Materials	Scent Character
Rose	Rose Otto, Rose, Geranium Rose, Palmarosa	rich, romantic, soft
Jasmine	Jasmine Sambac/ grandiflorum, Ylang Ylang, Tuberose	narcotic, exotic, sweet
Orange Blossom	Neroli, Petitgrain sur fleurs, Bitter Orange	bright, citrus-floral

Floral Note	Natural Materials	Scent Character
Lilac (reconstructed)	Jasmine, Ylang Ylang, Rose Geranium, Violet Leaf	springlike, delicate
Gardenia (reconstructed)	Tuberose, Jasmine, Coconut, Ylang Ylang	creamy, tropical floral
Violet	Violet Leaf Absolute, Orris Root, Mimosa	powdery, green-floral

Citrus Family

Citrus Note	Natural Materials	Scent Character
Bergamot	Bergamot FCF or expressed	green, sweet, lively
Lemon	Lemon, Lemon Myrtle, Litsea Cubeba	zesty, bright
Grapefruit	Grapefruit, Pink Grapefruit, Tagetes	tart, bitter-sweet
Orange	Sweet Orange, Blood Orange, Orange Essence	juicy, sweet, vibrant
Lime	Lime (distilled or cold-pressed)	sour, energizing

Woody Family

Woody Note	Natural Materials	Scent Character
Sandalwood	Santalum Album, Amyris, Spikenard	creamy, soft, sacred
Cedar	Atlas Cedarwood, Himalayan Cedar, Virginian Cedar	dry, pencil-shaving wood
Vetiver	Vetiver (aged), Patchouli, Oakmoss	earthy, damp, smoky
Oud /Agarwood	Oud, Agarwood, Patchouli + Birch Tar	animalic, resinous, mysterious

Gourmand Family

Gourmand Note	Natural Materials	Scent Character
Vanilla	Vanilla Absolute, Benzoin, Tolu Balsam, Tonka Bean	sweet, warm, dessert-like
Chocolate	Cocoa Absolute, Coffee, Vanilla	rich, edible, dark
Honey	Beeswax Absolute, Immortelle, Orange Blossom	syrupy, golden
Caramel	Benzoin, Labdanum, Peru Balsam	burnt sugar, buttery
Coffee	Coffee, Chicory Tincture	roasted, bold

Fresh/Oceanic Family

Fresh Note	Natural Materials	Scent Character
Marine/Aquatic	Seaweed Absolute, Cypress, Violet Leaf	salty, sea-breeze
Clean Linen	Lavender, Neroli, Geranium, Eucalyptus	soapy, airy, crisp
Rain/Ozone	Eucalyptus, Peppermint, Violet Leaf	wet, dewy, fresh air
Aldehydic Freshness	Litsea Cubeba, Lemon Myrtle, Citronella	sparkling, clean, sharp

Oriental/Resinous Family

Resinous Note	Natural Materials	Scent Character
Incense/Temple	Frankincense, Myrrh, Opoponax, Styrax	sacred, meditative
Amber	Labdanum, Vanilla, Benzoin, Cistus	sweet, warm, glowing
Leather	Birch Tar, Labdanum, Styrax	smoky, animalic, dark
Balsamic	Benzoin, Peru Balsam, Tolu Balsam, Elemi	sweet-resin, vanilla undertone

APPENDIX B
Famous Perfume Accords

Fragrance Name	Accords	Key Notes
Chanel No. 5 (Chanel)	Aldehydic, Floral, Woody	Aldehydes, Jasmine, Rose, Sandalwood, Vetiver
Shalimar (Guerlain)	Oriental, Vanilla, Citrus	Bergamot, Iris, Opoponax, Vanilla, Tonka Bean
J'adore (Dior)	Floral, Fruity, Sweet	Ylang Ylang, Rose, Jasmine, Pear, Melon
Opium (Yves Saint Laurent)	Oriental, Spicy, Woody	Clove, Myrrh, Jasmine, Amber, Opoponax
Light Blue (Dolce & Gabbana)	Citrus, Fruity, Fresh	Sicilian Lemon, Apple, Bamboo, Cedar, Amber
Angel (Thierry Mugler)	Gourmand, Sweet, Patchouli	Bergamot, Red Berries, Vanilla, Caramel, Patchouli
Coco Mademoiselle (Chanel)	Oriental, Citrus, Floral	Orange, Jasmine, Rose, Patchouli, Vetiver

Fragrance Name	Accords	Key Notes
La Vie Est Belle (Lancôme)	Sweet, Fruity, Floral	Blackcurrant, Pear, Iris, Praline, Vanilla
Black Opium (Yves Saint Laurent)	Oriental, Coffee, Vanilla	Coffee, Pink Pepper, Orange Blossom (Neroli), Jasmine, Vanilla
Miss Dior (Dior)	Floral, Citrusy, Woody	Italian Mandarin, Jasmine, Rose, Patchouli, Musk
Aventus (Creed)	Fruity, Smoky, Woody	Pineapple, Birch, Musk, Blackcurrant, Vanilla
Dior Sauvage (Dior)	Fresh, Spicy, Citrus	Bergamot, Sichuan Pepper, Lavender, Geranium, Vetiver
Flowerbomb (Viktor & Rolf)	Floral, Sweet, Powdery	Jasmine, Orange Blossom, Patchouli, Rose, Vanilla
Euphoria (Calvin Klein)	Woody, Fruity, Floral	Pomegranate, Persimmon, Black Orchid, Amber, Mahogany
Noir de Noir (Tom Ford)	Floral, Spicy, Sweet	Saffron, Black Rose, Truffle, Vanilla, Patchouli
Hypnotic Poison (Dior)	Vanilla, Almond, Powdery	Almond, Jasmine, Caraway, Vanilla, Musk
Allure Homme Sport (Chanel)	Citrus, Aquatic, Spicy	Orange, Sea Notes, Pepper, Neroli, Tonka Bean

Fragrance Name	Accords	Key Notes
Bleu de Chanel (Chanel)	Citrus, Woody, Spicy	Grapefruit, Lemon, Pink Pepper, Ginger, Sandalwood
L'eau d'Issey (Issey Miyake)	Aquatic, Floral, Fresh	Lotus, Freesia, Cyclamen, Musk, Cedar
Terre d'Hermès (Hermès)	Woody, Citrus, Earthy	Orange, Grapefruit, Pepper, Flint, Vetiver
Le Male (Jean Paul Gaultier)	Aromatic, Fresh, Vanilla	Mint, Lavender, Vanilla, Cinnamon, Amber
Light Blue Pour Homme (Dolce & Gabbana)	Citrus, Fresh, Spicy	Sicilian Mandarin, Juniper, Bergamot, Pepper, Musk
L'Instant de Guerlain (Guerlain)	Oriental, Woody, Floral	Lemon, Bergamot, Jasmine, Patchouli, Honey
Prada Amber Pour Homme (Prada)	Amber, Powdery, Woody	Cardamom, Neroli, Vetiver, Tonka Bean, Vanilla
Guerlain Homme (Guerlain)	Fresh, Woody, Aromatic	Mojito, Lime, Mint, Vetiver, Cedar

These accords are the core of each perfume's character and can be recreated with essential oils of similar profiles. You don't always use equal drops of each accord. The proportion of each accord depends on the desired final scent profile.

All-Natural Perfume Clone Recipes

These formulations recreate popular commercial perfumes using natural aromatic materials. The extraction method may vary depending on availability.

Chanel No. 5–Inspired (Classic Aldehydic Floral)

A classic floral perfume inspired by the aldehydic style, featuring bright, sparkling lift and a soft, powdery drydown, with aldehydic character interpreted through natural materials rather than synthetic aldehydes.

Style: Powdery, floral, refined

Note	Ingredient	Drops
Top	Lemon	4
	Bergamot	6
	Neroli	4
	Ylang Ylang	3
Heart	Jasmine	8
	Rose Otto	5
	Orris Root (diluted)	3
	Lilac Accord (natural floral blend)	4
Base	Sandalwood	6
	Vetiver	3
	Oakmoss	2
	Vanilla	3

Dior Sauvage-Inspired (Fresh Spicy Woody)

A fresh, spicy woody composition with a vibrant citrus opening, aromatic herbal heart, and a dry, mineral-leaning woody base designed to echo the clean, expansive character of the original fragrance.

Style: Crisp, modern, masculine

Note	Ingredient	Drops
Top	Bergamot	10
	Black Pepper	4
Heart	Lavender	6
	Geranium Bourbon	3
	Pink Pepper	2
Base	Amyris	4
	Sandalwood	4
	Labdanum	3
	Benzoin Resinoid (diluted)	2
	Cedarwood Atlas	5

Black Orchid-Inspired (Oriental Floral Gourmand)

A rich oriental floral gourmand with dark florals, warm spice, and a creamy, resinous sweetness, structured to feel opulent, dense, and slowly unfolding on the skin.

Style: Dark, exotic, unisex

Note	Ingredient	Drops
Top	Black Currant Bud	4
	Ylang Ylang	6
	Cocoa	2
Heart	Jasmine	5
	Lotus (natural floral blend)	3
	Orchid (jasmine + ylang + violet)	3
Base	Patchouli	8
	Frankincense	4
	Cacao	2
	Vanilla	4

Light Blue-Inspired (Citrus Fruity Woody)

A bright citrus fruity woody fragrance with a crisp, sparkling opening, a clean, lightly aromatic heart, and a smooth woody base that feels fresh, modern, and easy to wear.

Style: Sparkling, clean, daytime

Note	Ingredient	Drops
Top	Lemon	8
	Grapefruit	4
	Petitgrain	3
	Apple Accord (Roman Chamomile + Litsea)	3
Heart	Jasmine	4
	Bamboo Accord (Vetiver + Violet Leaf)	3
Base	Cedarwood Atlas	6
	Amyris	3
	Labdanum	2

***Aventus-Inspired* (Fruity Chypre)**

A bold fruity chypre structure combining a fresh, vibrant fruit opening with a smoky, woody heart and a dry, mossy base for a confident, modern character.

Style: Bold, smoky, modern masculine

Note	Ingredient	Drops
Top	Bergamot	8
	Blackcurrant Bud	3
	Pineapple Accord (Litsea + Chamomile + Ylang Ylang)	4
Heart	Birch Tar (sparingly)	1
	Jasmine	4
	Patchouli	3
Base	Oakmoss	3
	Labdanum	2
	Vanilla	3

Black Opium-Inspired (Gourmand Oriental)

A warm, gourmand oriental composition with sweet, creamy facets layered over soft florals and a deep, comforting base that feels rich, addictive, and enveloping.

Style: Sweet, cozy, evening wear

Note	Ingredient	Drops
Top	Pink Pepper	3
	Orange Blossom	4
	Coffee Extract or Tincture	2
Heart	Jasmine	4
	Anise (Licorice substitute)	1
Base	Vanilla	5
	Patchouli	4
	Cedarwood Atlas	4

La Vie Est Belle-Inspired (Fruity Floral Gourmand)

A soft, fruity, floral gourmand with bright fruit notes, a smooth floral heart, and a sweet, creamy base that feels elegant, comforting, and luminous.

Style: Feminine, radiant, modern

Note	Ingredient	Drops
Top	Pear Accord (Ylang Ylang + Lemon)	4
	Blackcurrant Bud	3
Heart	Jasmine	4
	Orange Blossom	3
	Orris Root (diluted)	3
Base	Vanilla	4
	Patchouli	3
	Balsam of Peru or Benzoin Resinoid	2

www.ingramcontent.com/pod-product-compliance
Lightning Source LLC
Chambersburg PA
CBHW070812280726
48660CB00015B/405